Sinusitis, Hay Fever, Allergic Rhinitis Explained

Symptoms, signs, treatment, remedies, relief, cure, natural remedies, prevention, home remedies, medicine, vaccine, and surgery all covered!

By: Frederick Earlstein

Copyrights and Trademarks

Disclaimer and Legal Notice

Foreword

While we can all agree that breathing is pretty fundamental to sustaining life, most of us don't realize just how comfortable it is to have nice, open sinus passages until we don't.

Sinus infections are, simply put, miserable. Pressure builds up in your face or forehead. You have a dull, thudding headache. You can't taste anything. You can't smell anything. You've got nasty, thick mucus draining down your throat.

At night you can't sleep, but you're so exhausted all day you're nodding off at your desk. Everyone has a theory about what will and won't fix the problem. You're just trying to live through it.

For most of us, this is an occasional event, maybe precipitated by a cold that turns into a longer sick spell. For some people, however, "sinusitis" is a regular occurrence that seems to defy all treatment.

These people are caught on an endless round of antibiotics. They buy enough over-the-counter medications to keep the pharmaceutical companies afloat single-handedly. Tissues come into the house by the case.

Many sinusitis sufferers become addicted to nasal sprays. If they don't get their "hit" every few hours, they can't breathe at all. What the heck is it? An infection? Hay fever? An allergy?

Foreword

In truth, any one or all of those things could be responsible for your ongoing misery. Throw a few environmental pollutants and the stray bit of fungi into the mix and you can be facing a veritable panoply of potential causes.

The first step toward managing sinusitis is simply to understand what's going on in your nose, nasal cavity, and sinuses. That's the primary purpose of this book – education.

All treatment for any illness or chronic condition should be based on informed consent. You can't make good decisions about how to care for your health if you don't understand what's going on with your body.

The text of this book looks at the structure of the human nasal passages before moving in progression through an examination of a simple sinus infection to chronic and stubborn cases caused by multiple factors.

Along the way, you'll learn the language your doctor will use with you and develop a general familiarity with the conventional and non-standard ways sinusitis and its related conditions including allergic rhinitis or "hay fever" are handled.

By the end of the book, your functional understanding of sinusitis should be considerably more extensive, and hopefully you will have gained insight into your own condition.

Foreword

While sinusitis can be a stubborn ailment, it is not necessarily "incurable," although you may find that you have to adjust your definition of "cure." Regardless, you should feel less at the mercy of a physical condition that, while not necessarily mysterious is often misunderstood.

Foreword

Acknowledgments

I would like to express my gratitude towards my family, friends, and colleagues for their kind co-operation and encouragement which helped me in completion of this book.

My thanks and appreciations go to my colleagues and people who have willingly helped me out with their abilities.

Acknowledgments

Table of Contents

Table of Contents

Table of Contents

Table of Contents

Table of Contents

Part 1 – What's Making Me Sneeze

The real problem with sinus "problems" is how easily the symptoms they cause are confused with those of the common cold or allergies (seasonal and environmental). Depending on which nasal cavities are involved, you might even be diagnosed with migraines.

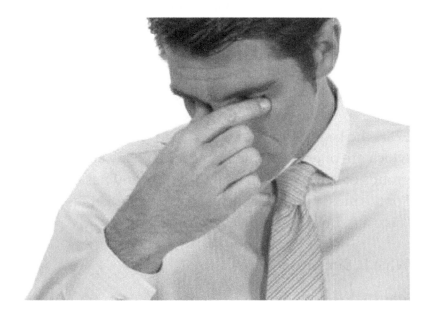

Long-term, chronic sinus problems adversely affect the lives of millions of people each year, causing pain, insomnia, fatigue, and an overall diminishment in the sufferer's ability to enjoy life.

Sinusitis causes people to limit their leisure activities, like playing sports, and it raises the potential for life-long addiction to nose sprays and other "remedies."

In the United States sinusitis is more common than heart disease. In 2004, the U.S. Centers for Disease Control and Prevention published a report indicating 35 million adults battle some degree of sinusitis every year, missing an aggregate 25 million workdays as a result.

At the same time, however, Americans dole out about $200 million annually on over-the-counter and prescription medications in an effort to get their sinuses back in good working order.

Sinusitis, Hay Fever and Allergic Rhinitis

From the beginning, it's important to clarify these terms, which are often used interchangeably. They all refer to groups of symptoms affecting the nose and nasal passages. For the most part, we will be using the blanket term "sinusitis," but let's look at each one in turn.

What is Sinusitis?

In the simplest terms, sinusitis is an inflammation of the sinuses. There is, however, nothing simple about a condition that, in its short-term, acute phase resolves in a few weeks, but as a chronic problem may exhibit symptoms that fall up and down a broad spectrum of sinus-related secondary illnesses.

Unlike the common cold, which is caused by a virus, the culprit in triggering a bout of sinusitis is a one or more bacterium present in the respiratory system.

Sometimes you will see this same condition referred to as rhinosinusitis since both the nose and sinuses are often affected.

Adults age 20-65 are the most likely population to be confronted with sinus problems. Sinusitis is no respecter of persons, however, occurring equally among men and women.

Hay Fever and Allergic Rhinitis

"Hay fever" is the common term for allergic rhinitis. When a person breathes in dust or pollen to which they are allergic, the mucous membranes in the eyes and nose become inflamed and itchy.

This results in a runny nose and watery eyes, which can occur seasonally when a particular plant is pollinating, or be present year round with the reaction dependent on exposure.

People with hay fever in the spring tend to be sensitive to tree pollens, while summer allergies are generally to grass and weeds. In the fall of the year, weeds and fungus spores are the culprits.

When hay fever seems to be a year-round constant, the allergens are typically things that are present indoors like dust, feather bedding, carpeting, or animal dander. Mold in damp areas like basements and bathrooms can also be to blame.

The Perfect Nasal "Storm"

Because hay fever or allergic rhinitis leads to an inflammation of the mucous membranes, these conditions cause swelling in the nasal cavity and sinuses.

When the openings of the nasal cavities become blocked, a breeding ground for bacteria is created and infection can set in. The reason these conditions are discussed together is because of this intimate – and miserable – relationship.

While allergy treatments won't cure a sinus infection, controlling allergies can stave off such an episode. Allergies aren't themselves infections, but they create one of the many doors through which infection can enter.

The Human Nasal System

To understand the nature of the problem, it's important to get a clear picture of how sinuses actually function in the human body.

We think of our nose as being our most prominent and obvious facial structure. It allows us to draw air into our lungs and to exhale carbon dioxide.

Most of us have some vague sense of where our sinuses are located, but little if any understanding of the intricate system involved in taking a single breath and preparing that air to reach the lungs in optimal condition.

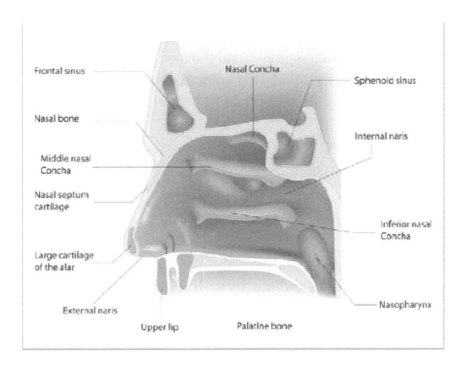

Frontal sinus
Nasal bone
Middle nasal Concha
Nasal septum cartilage
Large cartilage of the alar
External naris
Upper lip
Nasal Concha
Sphenoid sinus
Internal naris
Inferior nasal Concha
Nasopharynx
Palatine bone

Structure of the Nose

The human nose is comprised of a soft tip made of cartilage, and a hard bridge made of bone. In between is an area called the nasal valve, which collapses inward when we take a deep breath.

The width of the nasal valve varies from person to person, and can itself be the cause of breathing issues.

On the interior of the nose between each nostril there is a thin wall of flexible cartilage called the septum. It progresses 3-4 inches back into the head and becomes solid bone along the way.

Nasal Cavity

The nose leads to a region called the nasal cavity in which a series of openings called ostia adjoining four pairs of sinuses:

- maxillary - in the cheeks
- ethmoid - between the eyes
- frontal - in the forehead
- sphenoid - behind the nose

When the sinuses are healthy, the ostia are open, allowing air to flow freely in and mucus to drain out. If there is a problem, like swelling from an infection, the ostia close off and pressure builds up in the sinus.

The Turbinates

Humans can breathe through both their nose and mouth, but the nose is designed to both filter and warm the air we take in on its way to our lungs.

There are three sets of large bones behind the nose called the turbinates. The largest pair, the inferior turbinates, is at the bottom, roughly in a line with the base of the nostrils. They are approximately three inches in length.

On the next level up we find the slightly smaller middle turbinates (about 1.5 inches), and then the superior turbinates on top (an inch or less), roughly anterior to the bridge of the nose.

The turbinates circulate blood through their spongy, membranous surface to warm the air drawn in through the nostrils. Every six hours the volume of the blood flow in these surfaces switch sides as part of the nasal cycle.

If you have ever been aware of being able to breathe out of only one side of your nose, this is the normal functioning of the nasal cycle.

It switches back and forth throughout the day and night, but for the most part we are not aware of the change unless we consciously stop to check the air flow.

The air that comes into the nose and passes over the turbinates also picks up microscopic drops of moisture to improve its humidity level.

If you stand in front of a mirror and breathe on to the surface, the fog your breath creates illustrates the presence of this moisture in your nose.

Finally, the turbinates act as filters. The structures are covered in mucus that traps particles in the air we inhale and stops them from entering the lungs.

Ostiometal Complex

Before air reaches the sinuses, however, it must pass through the ostiomeatal complex, an area adjacent to the turbinates. Blockage of this structure is one of the most common triggers for an episode of sinusitis.

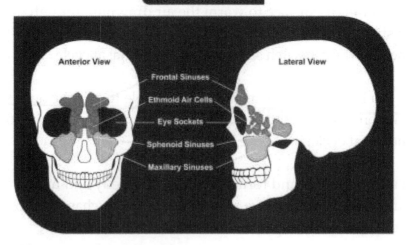

A Closer Look at the Sinuses

Pain and congestion can be present in each of the four pairs of sinuses or in combinations of these structures. This is why blocked ethmoid sinuses behind the eyes may be mistaken for a migraine, or issues with the maxillary sinuses may be wrongly diagnosed as a toothache.

Ethmoid Sinuses

The ethmoid sinuses are positioned between the eyes behind the bridge of the nose. They play a key role in the overall system of sinuses because the frontal and maxillary sinuses drain through them. If the ethmoids are not clear, the other sinuses will quickly become blocked as well.

The ethmoids are not single chambered, but are made up of 5-10 smaller chambers separated by thin walls covered with mucous membranes. The entire structure, however, is quite small, roughly the size of a matchbox.

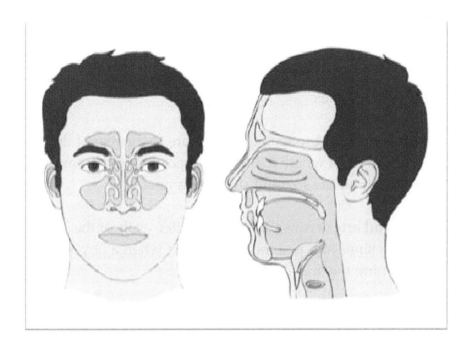

Maxillary Sinuses

The maxillary sinuses are located in the cheeks. If they sit low enough, the roots of the upper teeth extend into the cavity's floor. This is why some people experience upper tooth pain from a sinus infection.

The maxillary sinuses are triangular in configuration. Each one is roughly the size or a walnut.

Frontal Sinuses

If the frontal sinuses are present, they are located in the forehead between the eyes. About 90% of the population develops these sinuses.

The back wall of the frontal sinus is part of the bone that covers the brain. The size of the sinuses varies widely from person to person.

Sphenoid Sinuses

The deeply placed sphenoid sinuses are to the rear of the nose at the point where the eyes connect with the brain. They are about the size and shape of grapes.

The carotid artery runs through the outer walls of the sphenoid sinus and is sometimes visible when a physician is examining the area during surgery.

Internal Structure of the Sinuses

The surface of each of the sinus cavities is covered in small, bumpy glands that secrete mucus as well as a carpet of tiny hairs called cilia.

The sticky mucus serves to trap foreign particles and bacteria, while the cilia sweep the material away through the sinus opening and into the nose. The little hairs beat about six times a second and are very strong in relation to their size.

For instance, in order to push mucus through the ostia of the maxillary sinuses, the cilia actually have to overcome the force of gravity and move the material up to the opening.

This highly efficient process of mucociliary clearance moves approximately eight ounces of mucus a day through healthy sinuses.

Why Do We Have Sinuses?

In truth, there is no definite answer to the question of why human beings have sinuses. Without question, these empty spaces make the human head lighter, and thus may be an evolutionary adaptation to walking upright.

The structures also protect the eyes and brain by lessening the impact of blows to the face and head. They also make the structure of the skull less complicated so the facial bones can mature at an equal rate with the brain inside the cranial cavity.

These are not the only benefits derived from the sinuses, however. They improve our ability to taste and smell and provide resonance to the human voice.

The sinuses help to equalize pressure inside the nasal cavity and help to regulate our body temperature. Their filtering function is important to keep potentially harmful particles out of the lungs, and to ensure that the air we breathe is properly hydrated.

In fact, this whole system is a marvel of engineering efficiency as long as it's open and functioning. When something goes wrong, however, the consequences for the individual can be absolutely miserable.

In studies conducted at the Harvard Medical School, people with chronic sinusitis reported higher levels of ongoing pain and discomfort than those patients dealing with chronic neck and lower back pain and even heart disease.

What Causes Sinusitis?

There are many potential causes for sinusitis, but one of the most common is an obstruction of the ostiomeatal complex adjacent to the turbinate bones.

This causes mucus to back up into the sinuses, which shuts down the action of the cilia. The mucous glands, however, continue to do their job even though the "drain" is clogged.

Remember that the interior of the sinus is an area that is both moist and warm, making it a natural breeding ground for bacteria. Normally the bacteria that inhabit the area are perfectly safe.

However, when the sinuses back up and the mucus becomes stagnant and foreign debris is not being removed, harmful bacteria begin to rapidly proliferate until infection sets in.

Your Body's Response to Infection

Once that occurs, your body's defensive mechanisms are activated. The human immune response, which is attempting to protect you from the infection, is a large part of what makes you so miserable with full-blown sinusitis.

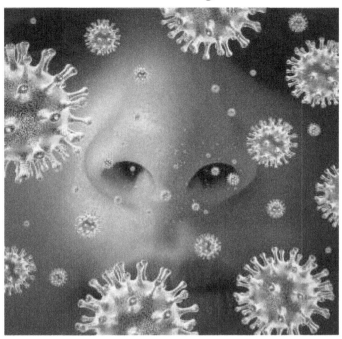

The mucous glands begin to work even harder, churning out vast amounts of mucus and swelling with blood to fight the bacterial invasion.

White blood cells rush to the membranous lining with the intent of destroying the bacteria. Basically your body has gone to war, and the battlegrounds are tiny spaces in your head that rapidly become filled to capacity.

The results are headaches, an awful feeling of pressure, thick mucus that sludges down the back of your throat, irritating the lining and causing even more discomfort.

You can't sleep at night. You can't concentrate by day. You feel awful. All because your body is doing exactly what it's supposed to do!

The longer the war goes on, the worse it tends to get. More of the sinuses become inflamed. There's more swelling, more blockage, more bacteria — welcome to the "sinusitis cycle." Now, what do you do about it?

Part 2 – Diagnosing and Treating Sinusitis

Although the symptoms of sinusitis are fairly straightforward, they can present concurrently with other conditions often leading to repetitive misdiagnosis.

Allergic rhinitis is one of those conditions. It is all too common for a doctor to put a patient through a round of allergy treatments that may, in fact, only serve to make their symptoms worse. If an infection is the underlying cause of the sinusitis, that must be addressed.

The more you understand about the often-stubborn sinusitis "complex," the more effectively you can participate in your own program of recovery.

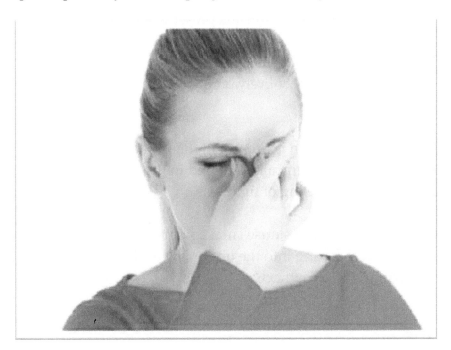

Major Sinusitis Symptoms

There are three major symptoms of sinusitis that make the condition often unbearable for the person suffering through a flare up.

- pressure / pain
- difficulty breathing due to congestion
- post-nasal drip / sore throat

Treating and resolving these symptoms is the challenge of breaking the sinusitis cycle.

Pressure and Pain

Pain from an attack of sinusitis presents with a throbbing, dull ache. Swelling in the inflamed sinus puts pressure on the nerve endings in the sinus lining. Where you feel the discomfort depends entirely on the location of the affected sinus.

- If the inflammation is present in the frontal sinus, you will have a headache, typically centered in the forehead with an accompanying feeling of tightness.

- Affected maxillary sinuses make your face hurt, with the pain often radiating into the upper jaw as if you were suffering from a toothache.

- When the condition strikes the ethmoid sinus the pain is in the bridge of the nose and between the eyes.

- Sphenoid sinuses cause pain behind the eyes and at the top and base of the head.

A single set of sinuses may be involved in an attack of sinusitis or all of the passages can be affected. If this is the case, the condition is referred to as pansinusitis.

Congestion and Difficulty Breathing

Over-production of mucus in combination with swollen membranes further narrows the breathing passages on one or both sides of the nose.

This congestion may just be an inability to draw air in freely, or it may be a painful sense of fullness and pressure. Some sinus sufferers say their head feels heavy or seems "too big."

If the ostia swell completely closed, the mucous membranes begin to absorb oxygen. This creates a vacuum which is even more painful.

Postnasal Drip and Sore Throat

Although mucus normally drains down the back of the throat, it is sufficiently thin that we don't notice it's there.

In the case of an infection, however, the mucus becomes thick and collects in the back of the throat, even pooling around the vocal cords.

This is why sufferers often wake up with a sore throat and a hacking cough until they can dislodge the mucus and cough it up.

High concentrations of white blood cells are present in this mucus, which irritate the lining of the throat. It is not at all uncommon for there to be excessive mucous discharge from the front of the nose as well.

Other Potential Symptoms

In addition to the three major symptoms of sinusitis, you may also experience:

- A diminished capacity to smell, which often accounts for the loss of appetite people experience during a bout of sinusitis.

- A concurrent lessening of the ability to taste. The human capacity to taste foods is dependent on smell. The loss of these two senses go hand in hand.

- Halitosis or bad breath caused by the bacteria present in the mucus drainage.

- Coughing as a measure to get rid of collected mucus in the back of the throat.

- Fatigue. In addition to the amount of energy your body is expending to fight the sinus infection, the symptoms of sinusitis make it almost impossible to get a good night's sleep.

- A sense of fullness in the ears due to blockages of the Eustachian tube, which connects to the ears to the back of the nose.

- A fever as part of the body's immunological response to the presence of the infection.

When people say that it's sometimes impossible to function well with a case of sinusitis, they are not exaggerating!

Difficulties in Diagnosis

The principle difficulty in diagnosing sinusitis is the similarity of symptoms to those present with colds and allergies. It is also possible for an attack of sinusitis to *begin* with either of these events.

The Common Cold and Allergic Rhinitis

It's important to realize that a virus causes the common cold, while bacteria triggers sinusitis. On average, a cold resolves in a week

Irritants in the environment cause allergies. They may be seasonal, or tied to instances of exposure to a substance to which the individual is sensitive (perennial).

Colds sometimes present with facial pressure and nasal discharge, but the mucus will be either thick and white or watery. If the mucus is from a sinus infection, it will be thick and greenish yellow.

Colds do not cause bad breath, but they do put the sufferer through coughing, sneezing, congestion, sore throat, and fatigue.

Nasal discharge from an allergy is clear, watery, and thin. Unlike either sinusitis or a cold, the person' eyes will itch. There will be no bad breath.

Sneezing will definitely be present, but congestion, coughing, and sore throat vary widely by individual.

In all cases, if the symptoms last for more than a week, a visit to your primary care physician is in order.

Visiting Your Doctor

When you see your doctor, the first step toward a diagnosis will be gathering information for a patient history. This process also involves excluding other conditions that might be responsible for your symptoms.

For instance, facial pain in the absence of congestion might indicate a neurological illness like neuralgia.

As a diagnostic tool, your doctor will look into the front of the nose using a small flashlight to illuminate the visible portions of the inferior turbinates to look for swelling and signs of infection.

Some doctors will tap on the forehead and cheeks looking for indications of tenderness, but this is actually not a reliable method to check for sinusitis.

X-Rays or CT Scan?

At one time, taking an x-ray of the sinuses was regarded as the most reliable test to determine the presence of sinusitis.

On an x-ray, bones show up as white, empty spaces as black, and other structures, including a sinus packed with mucous, appear in gray.

X-rays have been replaced by CT scans, however, as the best way to determine the presence of sinusitis.

CT scans use a series of x-rays that image 1-3 mm "slices," which are then assembled to give your doctor a 3D view of what's going on in your nose and sinuses.

The procedure is completely painless and quite fast, taking less than 5 minutes. There are two variations of the test: limited and full.

Of the two, a limited scan is less expensive and tends to be the type most often ordered by primary care physicians. For a simple case of sinusitis this test will be sufficient.

If, however, you are referred to an ENT (ear / nose/ throat) doctor with a particularly stubborn case of sinusitis, you will likely be asked to have a second, full scan performed.

This will allow the doctor to more thoroughly diagnose the cause of the ongoing discomfort.

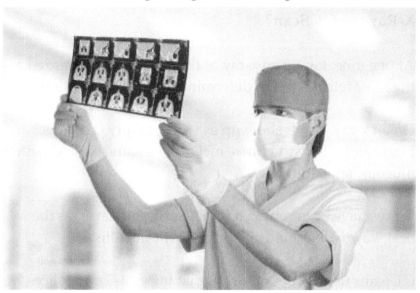

First Line Treatment

At the level of treatment you will receive from a primary care physician, you will likely be prescribed an antibiotic, and given advice on selecting an over-the-counter decongestant.

In a large number of cases, these measures will be sufficient to resolve an isolated case of sinusitis. If you have three or more episodes of sinusitis in any 12-month period, you will likely be referred to an ENT.

ENTs or otolaryngologists have specialized training and greater expertise in resolving persistent and chronic cases of sinusitis. Unlike primary care physicians, ENTs try to isolate the specific bacteria present, and look for and address physical abnormalities in the nasal cavity.

Referral to an ENT

If you are referred to an ENT, be prepared to go through your medical history again. Don't be impatient with this process. Every doctor needs to work his own diagnostic procedure and an ENT will likely ask much more detailed questions.

Endoscopic Examination

In all likelihood the doctor will start with a visual examination of your nose using a nasal speculum to gently widen your nostrils for better access.

Next, he may progress to an endoscopic exam using a high-resolution camera on a thin stem. The end of the instrument that enters your nasal cavity is lighted, and the opposite end is outfitted with an eyepiece through which the doctor views the area.

In preparation to insert the instrument, you'll receive a dose of a nasal decongestant spray and a mild topical anesthetic.

An endoscopic procedure doesn't hurt, but it does create a tickling sensation that makes it hard for the patient to sit still, which is necessary for the doctor to be able to get a good look inside your nose.

Using the endoscope, the doctor will look for inflammation of the mucous membranes and check the meatus for signs of infection and turbinate enlargement. It may also be possible for him to see any polyps that are further blocking the sinuses.

Nasal Polyps and Cysts

Both nasal polyps and cysts are quite commonly revealed during CT scans and endoscopic examinations. Neither is cause for undue concern.

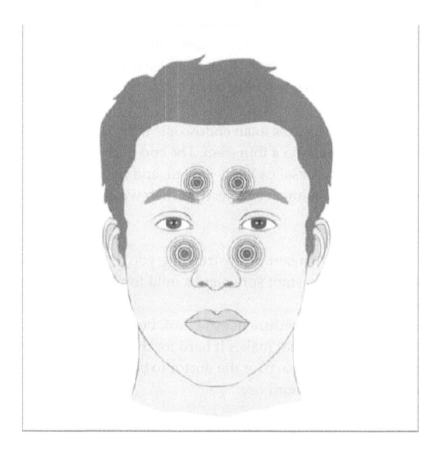

Cysts in the sinuses are filled with mucus and normally reach the size of a grape. They are typically quite harmless, and simply develop when a mucous gland becomes blocked.

Cysts occur most frequently in the maxillary sinuses.

When a cyst grows to its maximum size, it ruptures spontaneously and the mucus drains out. Most people have no idea this has even occurred, although they might notice a brief salty taste in their mouths. Very rarely does a cyst grow large enough that it requires surgical removal.

Polyps are growths roughly equal to the size of a pea. They grow on stalks emanating from the wall of the sinus and are common in people with chronically inflamed mucosa.

As the polyp grows, it can narrow the nasal passage causing congestion. Ultimately a polyp can completely block a sinus, triggering an overgrowth of bacteria and the development of sinusitis.

These growths rarely present as malignancies. It may be possible to shrink a polyp with the use of steroids, avoiding surgical removal.

Nasal Tumors

Any time a person is diagnosed with a growth of any sort, the mind naturally runs to one word "cancer." It's important to understand that nasal tumors are extremely rare. Polyps are not tumors.

When tumors do occur in the nasal passages, they are typically benign. Additionally, since the growths block the nose and cause sinusitis, they are detected early and easily removed.

If a nasal tumor was undetected, or allowed to grow quite large, it could certainly do a great deal of damage, but this rarely occurs.

Discovering Allergic Rhinitis

An endoscopic examination may also reveal swelling of the turbinates, especially the inferior turbinates. If this is the case, the greater sinus issue may actually be allergic rhinitis caused by environmental irritants that cause the nasal passages to swell.

Although the symptoms of allergic rhinitis are much the same as those of sinusitis, a CT scan may show that the sinuses are open.

Additional Testing

Depending on what your doctor sees through the endoscope, a full CT scan will likely be the next test ordered.

This could be followed by allergy testing or by a culture of the bacteria present in the nose. An MRI will not be ordered because an MRI works best to reveal details in soft tissue, not bony structures.

If a culture is performed, the swab will likely be taken using the endoscope again so the bacteria are obtained from the most seriously affected area. This will guide the doctor in prescribing the correct antibiotic.

Blood tests are also possible if your doctor believes that your sinus pain is linked to a larger systemic problem.

The Diagnosis

At this stage of combating your sinus problems, you will either be diagnosed with acute or chronic sinusitis. The only difference in the two labels is duration.

In a case of acute sinusitis, the symptoms resolve in 1-3 months. With chronic sinusitis, the symptoms last longer than three months.

Physiologically the only difference in the two diagnoses is that patients with acute sinusitis are more likely to have a fever.
If you are found to suffer from chronic sinusitis, you have a running battle on your hands, one where relapses are quite common.

Your quality of life will be affected to some degree, and finding the right combination of treatments to offer relief is more challenging.

Understanding Acute Sinusitis

In about 5% of cases, an episode of acute sinusitis is preceded by a cold. This progression is most likely in people who have naturally narrow sinus openings. During the cold, sinus drainage becomes impaired and the area swells, leading to a backing up of the mucus and a proliferation of bacteria.

Although the cold itself is caused by any one of several rhinoviruses, the secondary sinus infection will be touched off by one of three common bacteria:

- *Streptococcus pneumonia*
- *Haemophilus influenza*
- *Moraxella catarrhalis*

Typically, a secondary infection is more persistent and harder to "kick" than the original cold.

Treating Acute Sinusitis

Resolving a case of acute sinusitis while offering the patient some degree of physical relief involves the interplay of several treatment strategies.

Over-the-counter painkillers are useful for the headache and pressure that accompany a sinus infection. It doesn't really matter which product you choose. Acetaminiphen, ibuprofen, and aspirin will all work depending on personal preference.

Staying well hydrated is crucial. Getting as much water in your system as possible will help to thin the mucus in your sinuses for more effective and faster drainage.

This process should also include nasal irrigation with a saline solution, and exposure to steam from almost any source ranging from a comforting bowl of soup to a long, hot shower.

Ice compresses can also help with facial pain. Retail pharmacies sell special gel masks that can be frozen multiple times. These products are especially good because they conform more directly to the facial features for better coverage.

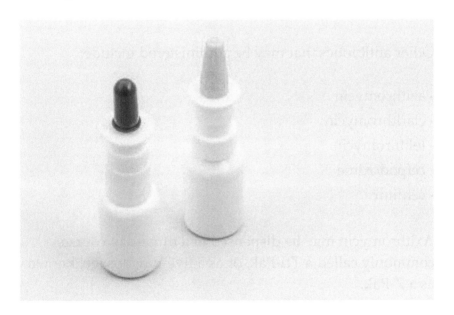

Prescription Medications

Once a patient is diagnosed with acute sinusitis, an ENT will prescribe an antibiotic and probably a decongestant. Although penicillin was once the standard treatment, too many strains of bacteria have developed resistance to the drug.

Antibiotics

Currently, amoxicillin is the most-prescribed medication, although it, too, is proving to be ineffective in as many as 30% of cases. The use of augmentin, a combination of amoxicillin and clavulanate is growing more popular for this reason.

Other antibiotics that may be administered include:

- azithromycin
- clarithromycin
- telithromycin
- cefpodoxime
- cefdinir

Axithromycin may be dispensed in a three-day course, commonly called a Tri-Pak, or as a five-day dosage, known as a Z-Pak.

The issue of decongestants is somewhat more complicated by how people use these medications on their own without a doctor's guidance.

The Problem with Decongestants

Both your primary care physician and your ENT may recommend that you use a decongestant in the form of either an over-the-counter spray or tablet.

If you have chosen not to see your doctor and are dealing with your sinusitis alone, seeking relief from the pressure and congestion is one of the first things you'll pursue.

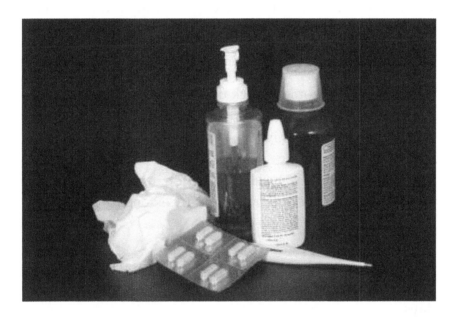

Nasal Sprays and Rebound

Nasal sprays offer one of the most direct and instant means of relief for painful sinus congestion – almost too quick. With over-the-counter medications, people often think that if one dose is good, two is better.

Part 2 – Diagnosing and Treating Sinusitis

Over-medicating with these items is common and dangerous. The implications for managing sinusitis are especially important.

The two active ingredients in most commercially available nasal decongestants are oxymetazoline or phenylephrine. Both cause a phenomenon called "rebound" if used for an extended period of time.

When rebound occurs, the swelling instantly returns when the effect of the spray wears off.

In fact, the swelling evident in rebound tends to be more severe, leading people to pick up the spray bottle and use even more of the preparation, seeking the same level of relief they initially received.

This sets up a vicious cycle of addiction, until the affected person literally cannot breathe for any extended period of time without a "hit" of nasal spray.

To avoid the development of rebound, a nasal spray with an active ingredient should never be used for more than 2-3 days.

A saline nasal spray can be used for any amount of time without fear of rebound, but these products do not deliver the same kind of dramatic results.

It is also a good idea to select a nasal spray that is formulated for mild doses of approximately four hours.

Regardless, only turn to a nasal spray to get yourself through really severe instances of congestion, otherwise, avoid these products.

Oral Decongestants

All oral decongestants have pseudoephedrine as their active ingredient. These pills are slower to provide relief from sinusitis, but they do not raise the potential for addictive rebound. They do, however, have other potentially harmful side effects.

People with high blood pressure should not use oral decongestants due to their propensity for causing heart palpitations.

Almost anyone can experience a sense of being "jittery" when taking pseudoephedrine, which can also cause insomnia.

Acute Sinusitis and Surgery

Thankfully in instances of acute sinusitis, surgery is almost never indicated unless the bacterial infection is so severe it actually breaks through a sinus wall.

If this were to occur, it would most likely happen in the ethmoid sinus where the intervening partitions are very thin.

Of those partitions, the lamina papyracea between the ethmoid sinus and the eye socket is the most vulnerable to perforations and abscesses.

Although rare, if this does occur, surgery is essential to drain the area and preserve vision.

Part 3 – The Challenge of Chronic Sinusitis

The greatest challenge of living with and treating chronic sinusitis is the variability of the problem. It is a mistake to think of sinusitis as a single condition.

Most experts are in agreement that chronic sinusitis presents on a spectrum or continuum with inconsistent responses to various treatments and forms of intervention.

No two cases are identical, making treatment even more challenging. The following milestones most often define the reference points on this spectrum:

- Patients whose nasal cavities and sinuses are affected by physical irregularities. This may include either a deviated septum or the presence of polyps.

- Individuals for whom sinusitis is one aspect of a broader problem affecting their entire system like allergic rhinitis or even an autoimmune disorder.

- People who have both a physical irregularity and a systemic problem.

- Those that have neither a physical irregularity nor a systemic problem, but still have sinusitis.

Since any gradation or combination of these factors is possible, chronic sinusitis can be an extremely difficult condition with which to deal.

Diagnosing Chronic Sinusitis

During the diagnostic process, doctors look for key signs that can indicate the root cause of the ongoing sinusitis. These factors may be present singly or in combination.

Physical Abnormalities

A critical part of diagnosing chronic sinusitis and developing a plan of treatment is determining if there are any physical irregularities present. These might include:

- an obstruction of the ostiomeatal complex
- enlarged turbinates (especially the middle turbinates)
- deviated septum
- an infected tooth adjacent to the maxillary sinus

If a physical abnormality is the cause of sinusitis, the following conditions may be present:

- symptoms localized to one side of the head or face
- no persistent symptoms like postnasal drop between infections
- no allergies detected via testing

Typically a person with sinusitis caused by a physical abnormality will experience good relief from medications, but once the treatment is stopped, all the problems return.

In these cases, surgery is generally indicated. The procedures can range from having a tooth removed to straightening the deviated septum. Recommendations for surgical intervention vary by individual case.

Chronic Inflammation

Chronic inflammation of the sinuses may also be present, extending to the mucous lining of the nose and even down into the lungs.

In about 30% of these cases, asthma is also a factor. If the same underlying cause is responsible for both the sinusitis and the asthma, the patient is said to have "one airway disease."

When mucous membranes in the sinuses are inflamed, polyps tend to form. These growths can cause significant congestion as they become larger. Often the polyps are present on both sides of the nose.

In severe cases, chronic inflammation leads to a triad of symptoms including asthma, polyps, and an allergic reaction to aspirin.

(About 10% of people with asthma have this combination, referred to as Samter's triad or aspirin-induced asthma.)

For sinusitis sufferers with chronic inflammation, symptoms may include:

- Congestion with an accompanying feeling of pressure on both sides of the face or head.

- Difficulty breathing through both sides of the nose without the intermittent relief of the normal nasal cycle.

- Thick and constant postnasal drip that is yellow or greenish in tint.

- A marked diminishment or complete loss of the sense of smell.

- Severe allergic rhinitis.

Cases of this type prove to be difficult to treat because even with the removal of the polyps, relief is only temporary. Oral steroids often work well, but cannot be used long term due to the side effects.

Combined Root Causes

People who have a combination of root causes underlying their sinusitis are often in for a frustrating course of diagnosis and treatment. They live in the land of "either / or" and "may or may not."

- They may have congestion on either one side or the other.
- Pressure may or may not accompany this congestion.
- One or more sinuses may be involved.
- They may or may not have severe allergies requiring treatment.
- Their flare-ups may or may not coincide with allergy season.

They will either have chronic inflammation or a physical obstruction including a deviated septum, enlarged middle turbinate, or polyps. Basically, people with combined root causes for their sinusitis are veritable grab bags of potential explanations.

Consequently, their symptoms may be equally variable:

- Alternating congestion.
- Intermittent thick and discolored postnasal drip.
- Symptoms improve but don't clear between infections.

A variety of treatment approaches will be necessary until the right combination is determined. No two people respond the same way to the treatment regimen.

Vacuum Sinusitis

Vacuum sinusitis is perhaps the most perplexing of all varieties of this condition. Patients complain of all the classic symptoms of sinusitis, but they have no infection and CT scans show their sinuses to be completely open.

One theory about this condition is that the ostia open and close intermittently. When the passage is closed, the sinus lining absorbs oxygen and a vacuum forms, which causes the pain and other symptoms.

Typically doctors will attempt to correct the condition with steroids and decongestants, and to look for other contributing factors, which could include neuritis, neuralgia, or migraines.

Fungus-Related Sinusitis

Cases of sinusitis related to the presence of fungus in the nose and sinuses remain somewhat controversial in the medical community.

Although fewer than 5 percent of sinusitis cases can be directly linked to fungi, in those instances, there are three types: fungus ball, allergic fungal, and invasive fungal sinusitis.

Fungus Ball

In fungus ball sinusitis, a literal "ball" of fungus grows inside the sinus passage, blocking the opening. In most cases the only way to eradicate the mass is with surgery.

The procedure has a very high rate of success and once the fungus is removed, it is rare for symptoms to recur.

Allergic Fungal Sinusitis

Allergic fungal sinusitis is a reaction to fungus in the nasal cavity that leads to inflammation and the production of very dark, intensely thick mucus called "mucin."

These cases often present with both polyps and a secondary bacterial infection. Treatment is typically a combination of steroid sprays and antibiotics.

Surgery is ultimately required to clear away the fungus, but there is a high probability that the problem will be recurrent.

Invasive Fungal Sinusitis

Cases of invasive fungal sinusitis are the most rare form and occur only in patients with severely compromised immune systems.

These cases could include individuals with HIV/AIDs, uncontrolled diabetes, transplant recipients, or chemotherapy patients.

The fungus invades the walls of the sinuses, moving into the blood vessels and underlying bone and potentially reaching the brain.

If caught early, the only course of action is radical surgery to remove diseased and dead tissue and the administration of aggressive antifungal medications via IV. Invasive fungal sinusitis can, however, prove fatal.

Treating Chronic Sinusitis

There are both surgical and nonsurgical strategies that are routinely used in cases of chronic sinusitis. Many of these can be used at home, and, if applied routinely as preventive measures, are reasonably effective.

Nasal Irrigation Methods

Nasal irrigation alternately referred to as nasal rinsing or lavage keeps the nasal cavity clear of excess mucus and potentially harmful irritants like mold, bacteria, and dust.

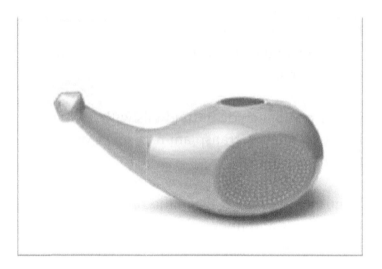

A popular method to accomplish this simple procedure is the use of a neti pot, which bears something of a resemblance to the sort of lamp a storybook hero might rub to produce a genie.

- Fill the pot with lukewarm, mild saltwater.
- The mixture is roughly 1 teaspoon per 8 ounces.
- Tilt the head sideways.
- Breathe through your mouth.
- Pour the water in the top nostril.
- The stream will wash through the nasal cavity.
- The water exits through the bottom nostrils.
- Reverse positions and repeat on the other side.

Salt water is used because mucus itself has a natural degree of salinity. If you poured plain water into your nose, it would sting horribly.

If you do experience discomfort, adjust the salinity mixture, or add about half a teaspoon of baking soda.

This easy procedure performed one or more times a day, can have near miraculous results for many people with chronic sinusitis. It is also a powerful preventive against sinus infections.

For those people who simply cannot get the hang of a neti pot, a plan bulb syringe used to clean out a newborn baby's nose will work as well. To use this method, lean over the sink with your head held slightly bowed.

The water will drain out the same nostril, or in some cases down your throat. Either is fine.

Whether you use a neti pot or a syringe, it's perfectly normal to feel the urge to blow your nose afterwards, and to get rid of mucus in the process.

There are motorized devices available for nasal irrigation. These are add-on attachments used with machines that are primarily intended to clean debris out from around the teeth and gums.

The stream of water from devices of this type is obviously more forceful, and may be best for people dealing with thick mucus that crusts in the nostrils overnight.

Thick mucus will also respond to the addition of a thinning agent in the water. Mucus thinning products are available at pharmacies and online. They are most often mixtures of several agents including, but not limited to:

- baking soda

- alcohol

- camphor

- menthol

- eucalyptus

It may be necessary to play with the mixture to get a version that does not sting the nasal passages. Start with whatever the box recommends, and dilute with lukewarm water as needed.

Home Humidifiers

Since most of us are in a constant state of mild dehydration anyway, lack of humidity in the home plays a leading role in worsening sinusitis symptoms by causing mucus to thicken even more.

During the winter, home heating systems suck even more moisture out of our environment. Humidity levels will drop to 20-30% over the recommended 40-50% for maximum comfort and health.

A basic humidifier, which costs less than $50 / £31, placed near the head of your bed at night replaces much of this moisture and will help you to wake up less congested.

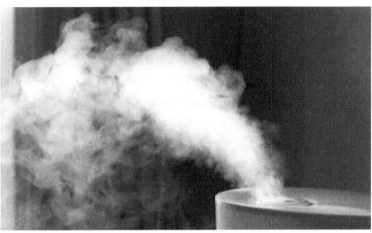

When using a humidifier, however, it is crucial that the device be kept clean or it will become a breeding ground for the very types of bacteria you are trying to keep out of your nasal passages.

It does not matter in terms of benefit if you opt for a cold or warm mist humidifier. The latter units, however, boil the water to produce steam, which helps to cut down on bacteria that may proliferate in the humidifier itself.

Nasal Tapes or Strips

Nasal tapes that are placed just above the bulge of the nostrils are useful in people who have a narrow nasal valve. This is the portion of the nose that moves inward as we breathe.

The strip is a simple measure to keep the nose more open at night. For sinusitis sufferers who have a deviated septum or who have suffered a broken nose at some point in their lives, nasal tapes often work very well.

Saline, the Safe Nasal Spray

Saline nasal spray should have a prominent place in the chronic sinusitis sufferer's arsenal of therapeutic options. Really for any form of inflammation of the nose, called simply rhinitis, saline sprays are comforting and effective.

The solution gently loosens accumulated thick mucus, even that temporarily caused by dry conditions like a long airplane flight.

There is no danger of rebound with a saline solution, and the spray can be used as often as you like.

The sprays come in both plain and augmented versions that include additional soothing and decongesting agents like camphor and eucalyptus. All of these substances are natural, safe, and not addictive.

Cold and Allergy Medications

The major caution in using over-the-counter cold and allergy medications is to use them sparingly in combination and then only to match your existing symptoms. The categories of OTC items for use with sinusitis include:

- decongestants
- cough medicine
- mucus thinners
- antihistamines
- painkillers

All are intended as methods of symptom relief, although none constitute a "cure." If you do opt for a single medication with multiple active agents, try to find the combination that best matches your current symptoms. Don't take anything you don't need.

Decongestant Sprays and Pills

With decongestant sprays, you will encounter products with one of two active ingredients, oxymetazoline or phenylephrine. Both carry a serious potential for nasal rebound and should not be used for more than three days.

The primary decongestant pill is pseudoephedrine, which reduces blood flow to the mucous membranes thus lowering levels of swelling. This medication, however, causes elevated blood pressure, heart palpitations, and insomnia. Patients who also have hypertension should not use it.

Cough Medicine

The most common cough medicine sold over the counter uses dextromethorphan as an active ingredient. It is available in both day and night time formulations.

Typically a cough suppressant is only required when there are significant amounts of mucus draining into the back of the throat. Often people with sinusitis cough at night because their body is trying to expel this pooled mucus.

Mucus Thinners

The only mucus thinning agent available is guaifenesin. It is very effective and produces fast relief. When using a mucus thinner, however, it's important to drink more than the normal amount of water as the drug must have water to deliver maximum relief.

Antihistamines

Often doctors recommend against the use of antihistamines, which tend to dry out the nasal passages even more. Many patients find, however, that antihistamines do make them feel better, so there is little harm in giving one of these medications a trial run.

The major antihistamines on the market include:

Sedating

- chlorpheniramine
- dramine
- bromphenirmaine
- clemastine

Non-Sedating

- loratadine
- desloratadine
- fexofenadine
- cetirizine

Sprays

- azelastine

Azelastine spray does not carry the danger of rebound, but it is not as effective as an oral antihistamine and users report that it tastes awful.

Painkillers

A word of caution; often cold and allergy medications also include a pain reliever in combination, so make sure you're not double dosing yourself!

The primary choices for painkillers are:

- aspirin
- acetaminophen
- ibuprofen
- non-steroidal anti-inflammatories

Any of these preparations are fine. Individuals respond to each one differently, so pick the medication that best relieves the headache and pressure.

Prescription Corticosteroids

Corticosteroid sprays are prescribed to treat inflammation in the sinuses and to shrink nasal polyps. These drugs are typically used first in an effort to avoid surgery.

The spray delivers the medication directly to the nasal membranes in high concentration, which greatly increases the intended benefits.

If a steroid spray is going to be effective, improvement will be seen in four to five days. Interestingly, however, although there is no scientific evidence that any one steroid works better than another, patients will inexplicably respond to one brand over another.

It's important to understand this fact. If your doctor gives you one steroid that does not work, do not rule out trying a second or even a third spray.

These medications, when used as directed, don't have long-term negative effects like those seen in the anabolic steroids used in excess by some athletes.

Potential mild side effects include both nosebleeds and an uncomfortable burning. However, once you have learned to deliver the spray with the nozzle directed toward the outside of the nose and not against the septum, both of these issues will disappear.

Used once a day, a steroid nose spray can provide significant relief, and can help a chronic sinusitis sufferer with polyps avoid nasal surgery.

Oral Steroids

If nasal steroids do not work for you, there are two oral varieties, prednisone and methylprednisolone. Both can be effective in lessening postnasal drip and opening congested passages within 24 hours of the initial dose.

These drugs also work to reduce polyps, but they should not be used for long periods of time due to the potential side effects, which include:

- weakened bones and potential osteoporosis
- thinning of the skin with excessive bruising
- diminished immune response
- cataracts
- stomach ulcers
- fluid retention

When oral steroids are used, the prescription is usually for a short course of a week or less. Doctors advise patients that they should not use oral steroids more than three times in one 12-month period.

Antibiotics in Detail

As was discussed in Part 2, amoxicillin is the most-prescribed medication for acute sinusitis even though it is ineffective in 30% of cases.
Many of the bacteria responsible for sinus infections have already developed immunity to the drug.

Doctors are now opting to dispense augmentin, which is a combination of amoxicillin and clavulanate. currently, this drug is proving effective, but over time, and due to patients who do not finish the prescribed course, too, will likely become ineffective.

Part 3 – The Challenge of Chronic Sinusitis

When these drugs do not work to fight sinusitis, your primary care physician will begin to run through the other available options one at a time. These drugs include:

- azithromycin
- clarithromycin
- telithromycin
- cefpodoxime
- cefdinir

Axithromycin is available as a Tri-Pak (three-day dose) or as a Z-Pak (five-day course.)
In chronic cases of sinusitis, your ENT will be somewhat more aggressive in using antibiotics in an attempt to eliminate the specific bacteria causing the infection.

When an initial course of antibiotics fails to kill the infection, the next step is to try a broad-spectrum variety for a long course of three weeks or more.

Chronic cases of sinusitis are often "polymicrobial," with two or more bacteria responsible for the essential war being waged behind your clogged ostia.

Culturing Bacteria

When cultures are taken, the bacteria most commonly seen in cases of chronic sinusitis are:

- *Staphylococcus aureus*
- *Pseudomonas*

- *Klebsiella*
- *Peptostreptococcus*
- *Fusobacterium*
- *Bacteroides*
- *Escherichia coli*

Using an endoscope, your ENT will take a small sample of mucus or pus from the area around the infected sinus, which will be incubated over a period of 5-7 days in the lab in an effort to isolate the bacteria present.

Selecting an antibiotic based on the results of the culture is the best option for finding an effective treatment without a lot of "hit and miss" efforts.

Classes of Antibiotics

Your doctor will have four classes of antibiotics from which to choose a treatment. These include:

- penicillins
- cephalosporins
- macrolides
- quinolones

Penicillins are rarely prescribed, however, as too many types of bacteria are now resistant to these older medications. Amoxicillin, which is a variant of penicillin, is also becoming less and less effective.

When sinusitis does not respond to amoxicillin, the next class of antibiotics typically used is the cephalosporins:

- cephalexin
- cefdinir
- cefixime
- cefpodoxime
- cefuroxime

They are effective in 90% of sinus infections caused by *Staphylococcus aureus*. The cephalosporins are also the drugs usually prescribed after sinus surgery.

For patients that are allergic to amoxicillin, macrolides are typically used:

- erythromycin
- azithromycin
- clarithromycin
- telithromycin

The quinolines are broad-spectrum antibiotics that effectively fight gram negative bacterias like *Pseudomonas*.

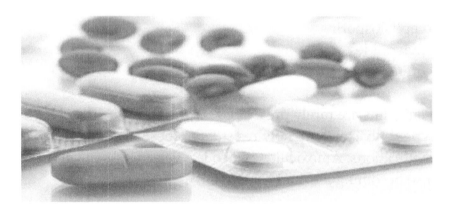

These are the antibiotics typically used with sinusitis when all of the others have failed to provide relief. The quinolines include:

- ciprofloxacin
- gatifloxacin
- levofloxacin
- moxifloxacin

There are, however, a range of potential side effects that can result from the use of powerful, broad spectrum antibiotics, including, but not limited to:

- an allergic reaction in 5-10 percent of cases
- gastrointestinal distress
- yeast infections in women
- a hypersensitive reaction to sunlight

Broad spectrum antibiotics can also interact negatively with other medications being used, a potential that should be explored fully with both your doctor and your pharmacist.

Women who are pregnant or nursing should not take broad-spectrum antibiotics without first consulting with their obstetrician or pediatrician.

The Decision to Have Surgery

The decision to have any kind of surgery should always be a matter of informed consent. You need to know everything about the potential procedure and its possible outcomes, both good and bad before moving forward.

Simply being frustrated with a long battle against chronic sinusitis is not sufficient reason to submit to an invasive procedure with no guarantee of success.

Your Doctor's Recommendation

Your doctor will make the recommendation for surgery based on a number of factors including:

- How many sinus infections you have per year.

Some people have so many infections in a 12-month period they never really reach a state of being "well." At that point in time, the effect of the sinusitis on the overall quality of life and general health must be considered.

- The duration of each infection.

Granted, you may only have three sinus infections a year, but if each one is lasting three months, you're not getting much relief. This can have just as negative an impact on your life as multiple infections.

The Decision is Yours

In the end, however, the decision is yours. Sinusitis is not life threatening. The surgery is elective, meaning it's your choice. You'll need to ask yourself some probing questions and be honest about the answers:

- Are you losing so much sleep you have chronic fatigue?
- Are you missing a large number of work days?

- Are you tired of taking medication constantly?
- Are you missing out on activities you enjoy?

Some people have a capacity to put up with almost anything, while others are easily worn down by the repetitive and unpleasant cycle of chronic sinusitis.

Consider Personal Risk Tolerance

You also have to consider your personal risk tolerance and determine what would be an acceptable outcome in your mind from a surgical procedure.

It's highly unlikely you'll be "cured." It may simply be that you go from 3 sinus infections a year to 2. Is that enough of a benefit in your mind?
Also, are you prepared for the potential of complications? These might include bleeding, infection, and even a worsening of your symptoms.

While the greater symptoms only occur in about five percent of cases, it is possible to lose your sense of smell after sinus surgery, to have even more trouble breathing, and to experience over-production from the tear ducts.

Minimally Invasive Procedure

Unlike the sinus surgeries that were performed 25 years ago, the modern procedure, functional endoscopic sinus surgery (FESS), is much less physically and emotionally traumatic.

All work is done through an endoscope, generally as a day surgery under a local or general anesthetic, with no external bruising.

Typically the surgeon will:

- Open the osteomeatal complex to inspect the maxillary sinuses for proper drainage.

- Enlarge the opening to the maxillary sinuses by removing obstructions, which might include polyps or swollen mucous membranes.

- Take out the partitions that separate the chambers of the ethmoid sinus and possibly excise diseased tissue from this region.
It may also be necessary to realign a deviated septum, and cultures may be taken of all these areas to pinpoint what bacteria might be thriving in the nasal cavity.

Advanced Sinus Surgeries

More advanced surgical work on the sinuses could include any of the following procedures:

- Sphenoid Sinusostomy: Enlarging the sphenoid ostia to allow for better fluid drainage. This is a delicate surgery due to the proximity of the sphenoid sinus to the optic nerve and brain.

- Frontal Sinusostomy: An enlargement of the ostia of the frontal sinus. This procedure is complex due to the location of the sinuses in the forehead requiring the use of specialized curved instruments.

- Frontal Sinus Drillout: The removal of the floor of the frontal sinus to create a large opening to maximize drainage.

- Frontal Sinus Obliteration: This surgery requires an incision in the forehead or through the scalp. All tissue inside the frontal sinus is removed and the space is filled with fat tissue removed from the abdomen. This seals the sinus, preventing the cavity from being infected in the future.

New advancements in sinus surgery now allow doctors to work with image-guided technology, greatly enhancing the accuracy of any of these procedures.

Recovering from Sinus Surgery

Modern sinus surgeries typically do not leave the patient with a great deal of pain, but you will likely feel very tired for a few days, and potentially experience a dull headache.

The mucus that drains from the nose will be bloody, but that should subside after a day or two. You may or may not come home with your nose packed in gauze, depending on how much you've bled during the procedure itself.

Nasal congestion following surgery is perfectly normal since your nasal cavity and sinuses will be more swollen from the trauma of the operation. You should not blow your nose for at least three days, but will rather be directed to irrigate with saline solution to keep your nose clear.

Any abnormal symptoms like bleeding, or developing a fever should be reported to your doctor immediately. Also report mucus with a green tint, and any severe facial pain.

For a week after surgery you will not be allowed to lift heavy objects or to strain in any way. In the second week you can gradually return to more normal daily activities, but limit exercise to slow walks.

Most people return to work in the second week and do well, other than reporting a tendency to tire more quickly. Drink plenty of fluids to stay well-hydrated. Driving is fine within 2-3 days after the procedure, but you should not take any airline flights for at least two weeks.

Expect a postoperative check-up a week to ten days after the surgery, followed by additional appointments as required by your doctor. Do not resume taking any medications until instructed to do so by your doctor.

Within one month, the swelling from the surgery will have gone down, but your body will not heal completely for 8-12 weeks. It could be several months before you can determine the full benefit of the procedure.

As difficult as it is to be patient, do not rush to assume that your sinus surgery has been a failure. It takes a while to judge just what kind of improvement you have gained.

Second or "Revision" Surgeries

In less than 5 percent of cases, it may be necessary for a second or "revision" surgery to be performed. Most often this is to remove scar tissue that has caused a new area of blockage.

These secondary procedures tend to be quite simple and require little more than a local anesthesia. If, however, the scar tissue is deep seated, the doctor may recommend a general anesthesia.

Part 4 – Lifestyle and Alternative Therapies

Although nutrition is still not being taught in medical schools as a primary course of intervention against common illnesses, there is a direct link between diet and other lifestyle choices and sinusitis.

The Link to Food Allergies

When a persistent postnasal drip with morning accumulations of phlegm or mucus in the back of the throat is the primary symptom of sinusitis, food allergies should be strongly considered as the underlying cause.

Allergies to both milk and wheat stimulate the production of excess mucus and postnasal drip. Over time, the ostia leading into the sinuses will become blocked due to chronic irritation, and the stage is set for an infection to develop.

Testing for a potential food allergy works best by process of elimination. Stop consuming the items for 2-4 weeks and watch for signs of improvement. Be strict during the trial. Do not eat any foods containing either dairy or wheat.

If these items are the offending agents in the sinusitis cycle, improvement is often fast and dramatic.

Sinusitis and Alcohol

People with chronic sinusitis often experience a flare up of symptoms or develop a new infection approximately 24 hours after drinking alcohol. These individuals are reacting to impurities in the beverage called cogeners.

As a by-product of fermentation, cogeners improve alcohol's aroma and flavor, but they have properties similar to histamines. Sensitive individuals react with congestion, drainage, and sinus headaches.

If you believe you have this sensitivity, drink white wine, not red, and choose clear liquors like vodka or gin. Avoid dark beers as well.

Sinusitis and Tobacco

Obviously smoking tobacco has an adverse effect on your entire respiratory system. In relation to the sinuses in particular, the smoke damages the tiny cilia and hinders their ability to efficiently remove mucus and debris.

Smokers with chronic sinusitis will see dramatic improvement in their symptoms by stopping their consumption. While this may be a very difficult process, the benefits in terms of overall health are enormous.

Alternative Sinusitis Therapies

Particularly in cases of chronic sinusitis that have proven resistant to all the conventionally accepted therapies, alternative approaches should be considered so long as they do no additional harm.

Individuals respond differently to all types of treatment. Since the goal is primarily symptom relief, try alternative therapies, but talk to your doctor about what you're doing. The alternative treatment needs to be evaluated in the broader context of your medical condition.

Research all herbal supplements and check with your doctor and pharmacist to guard against negative interaction with prescription medications you are taking.

Use alternative treatments as a corollary to your regular treatments. Never stop a course of treatment without consulting with your doctor. This is especially important when using antibiotics.

Acupuncture

In traditional Chinese medicine, disruptions in the flow of the body's energy or "chi" are believed to be the cause of disease and illness.

Using fine, sterile needles, acupuncture therapists work with pathways in the body called meridians to re-establish proper flow or the chi and open blockages.

Chronic sinusitis patients who seek acupuncture therapy often get good relief from their associated facial pain and headaches. Some also report less congestion and drainage.

Part 4 – Lifestyle and Alternative Therapies

Herbs

There is considerable debate over the effectiveness of herbal remedies for almost any condition. It's important to understand that pharmaceutical manufacturers have a deep-set influence on the practice of medicine.

These companies make enormous profits from the drugs they sell, and therefore have a vested interest in disparaging natural remedies.

Typically when you read up on an herbal therapy the best-case conclusions you will find from conventional medical sources describe the results of studies on the use of the preparation as "mixed" or they may say "more research is needed."

So long as the herb will not interfere with other medications you are taking, and there are no other adverse side effects, there is no harm in trying. The most popular herbs used in cases of chronic sinusitis include:

- Echinacea, which may strengthen the immune system to ward off infections while lessening the duration and severity of an existing infection.

- Goldenseal, which reportedly has both antibacterial and anti-inflammatory properties.

- Bromelain, which is believed to reduce inflammation and thus lessen congestion and mucus discharge.

If you are contemplating sinus surgery, discuss all supplements you are taking with your doctor. Some of these preparations can increase bleeding and should be discontinued in advance of a surgical procedure.

Vitamins and Minerals

The two nutritional supplements most commonly used to combat sinus infections are Vitamin C and zinc. Popular and "official" opinions differ on this practice.

Studies insist that there is no real effect of taking large doses of Vitamin C to lessen the duration and severity of an episode, but many sinus sufferers swear by the practice.

Zinc, on the other hand, has been proven effective in shortening an infection if taken within 24-hours of the appearance of symptoms.

The Role of Stress in Sinusitis

Stress has a negative effect on all of the body's systems, and is especially detrimental in worsening chronic conditions like sinusitis.

Medical science is universal in the assertion that finding viable ways to relieve stress is beneficial to your overall health and wellbeing.

Methods of stress reduction vary widely by individual. Some people are relaxed by sitting meditation practices, which have been found to lower blood pressure and improve circulation.

Others break out in hives at the very thought of meditating and opt for a more active discipline like yoga or tai chi. It doesn't matter if you find stress-relief in mediating or jogging, the point is to do something to take the edge off modern life.

While none of these things will necessarily "cure" your sinusitis, they will relax your body, strengthen your immune system, and increase your ability to cope with the discomfort of your chronic condition.

Stress reduction techniques should be a major component of anyone's personal health care plan, and are easily used in combination with all other forms of therapy.

Part 5 – Frequently Asked Questions

The Basics

What purpose do sinuses serve?

Sinuses are basically pockets of air strategically located around the nasal cavity to facilitate airflow and to condition the air we breathe before it reaches the lungs.

In an evolutionary sense, they lighten the skull and lend resonance to the human voice while cushioning blows to the skull, especially in the area around the eyes.

The mucus and cilia inside the sinuses capture and remove impurities.

What are cilia?

The tiny hairs inside the sinuses that beat in a wave-like fashion six times per minute are called cilia. Their function is to remove mucus from the sinus chambers through the opening called the ostia.

If this opening becomes blocked, however, the cilia can't do their job. This problem is compounded in smokers because the tobacco smoke paralyzes the cilia.

If the sinus opening is blocked, why can't the cilia move the mucus?

Basically as the sinus cavity fills up with mucus, the area becomes a breeding ground for more and more bacteria. This thickens the mucus, which essentially drowns the cilia preventing them from moving.

Why can't I just breathe through my mouth?

You can breathe through your mouth, but that is more or less an emergency backup system. The nose conditions the air that is brought into the lungs, making it warmer and moister while filtering out debris and unwanted particles.

What causes sinusitis?

Sinusitis is most typically caused by a blockage in a part of the nose called the ostiomeatal complex. This causes mucus to back up in the sinus cavity creating a climate ripe for the proliferation of bacteria.

When enough bacteria are present for this closed space to become infected, the body's immune response kicks in, creating even more mucus production along with swelling.

Although the body is trying to protect you from the invading bacteria, this chain reaction of events makes all the symptoms of sinusitis worse. If the cycle is unchecked, the condition can become chronic.

Acute Sinusitis

Is sinusitis common?

Sinusitis is extremely common and is thought to affect about 30% of the population at any given time.

The condition often follows a bout of the common cold, extending the period of illness by as much as three weeks.

If sinusitis symptoms linger past three months, the problem then becomes "chronic."

Are instances of sinusitis increasing?

This is a difficult question to answer. Certainly pollutants in the air and ozone can make sinus problems much worse, so in major cities where air quality has been severely compromised there may be more cases of sinusitis as compared to a more rural region.

However, since allergies can also aggravate sinus issues, this comparison might not hold up to vigorous study.

How is sinusitis diagnosed?

Diagnosing sinusitis can actually be quite difficult since the symptoms are so similar to those of the common cold and allergies.

A careful medical history is important, as is some examination of the nose and nasal cavity. This will differ by the type of doctor consulted.

A primary care physician will likely use a nasal speculum to slightly enlarge the nostrils and then view the interior of the nose aided by a light.

An ENT, on the other hand, might use an endoscope, which is a small camera. This is an in-office procedure with a mild topical anesthetic applied to forestall any discomfort or "tickling" when the scope enters the nose.

CT scans could be ordered by either physician, although a primary care doctor is more likely to order a partial version of the test and an ENT a full scan.

(Regular X-rays are no longer considered a gold standard imaging test for this condition and MRIs are not effective for diagnosing sinusitis.)

Are symptoms of sinusitis worse in the morning?

Yes, people with sinusitis are more uncomfortable in the morning because mucus has pooled at the back of the nose and throat and even around the vocal cords overnight.

You may wake up with a sore throat and need to cough the mucus up out of your throat to be more comfortable as the day begins.

Often patients say warm or cold drinks help to soothe their throat and clear the irritation, which may or may not be present the remainder of the day.

Is the treatment period for sinusitis long?

The duration of treatment depends entirely on the severity of the sinusitis and on any complicating conditions like nasal polyps or even potential abscesses.

Typically acute sinusitis resolves in about three weeks, but can go on for as long as three months at which point the condition is termed "chronic."

Can any doctor treat sinusitis?

Any primary care physician is capable of diagnosing and treating a case of acute sinusitis, but in instances of chronic sinusitis (symptoms lasting more than 3 months), you will likely be referred to an ENT.

Which antibiotics are used to treat sinusitis?

Penicillin used to be the drug of choice for cases of sinusitis, but too many strains of bacteria are now resistant to that drug. In most cases the first antibiotic prescribed is amoxicillin , although it, too, is ineffective in about 30% of cases.

A newer drug, augmentin, which combines amoxicillin and clavulanate is growing in popularity. Other antibiotics that may be prescribed include:

- azithromycin
- clarithromycin
- telithromycin
- cefpodoxime
- cefdinir

What is the usual length of the course of antibiotics?

Generally a 10-day course of amoxicillin is the first line of treatment in a case of sinusitis, but extended treatment may be necessary if there is no significant improvement.

A doctor will switch you to another antibiotic, for instance augmentin, for an additional ten days. Depending on the level of response, it is not unusual for some form of antibiotic to be administered over a period of 6-8 weeks.

What other treatments are used in conjunction with antibiotics?

Your doctor will likely suggest that you use a decongestant in concert with the antibiotic to encourage the sinuses to drain and to relieve the sense of fullness and pressure that accompany sinusitis.

Decongestants come in both pill and spray form. It's important not to use a nasal spray for more than 3 days or you run the risk of the phenomenon of rebound.

When this happens, the swelling in the sinuses returns after the effect of the spray wears off and is generally even more pronounced.

Rebound leads to a dependence on nasal sprays that can be tough to kick. There is no problem with rebound in pills, but these medications can often cause heart palpitations and a "jittery" feeling as well as contributing to insomnia.

Are antihistamines used in the treatment of sinusitis?

The major argument against using antihistamines in a case of sinusitis is their effect in drying out the sinuses and further trapping bacteria in the chamber.

The goal in treating sinusitis is to restore the normal daily flow of mucus. On a daily basis, about 8 ounces of mucus is pushed out of the sinuses by tiny hairs called cilia. This material drains harmlessly down the throat.

Allergies can be present concurrently with sinusitis, however, which may indicate a need to use antihistamines. This is one of those gray areas of chronic sinusitis treatment.

Antihistamines may make you feel better initially by reducing the feeling of fullness and pressure, but they're not recommended for long-term use for sinusitis and they won't actually cure the symptoms.

With chronic cases, however, your doctor may try several combinations of medications to arrive at the right mix to relieve your particular symptoms.

Why does my doctor want to culture the bacteria in my nasal cavity?

Sinusitis can be caused by several strains of bacteria. Typically, however, the three that are the most likely culprits are:

- *Streptococcus pneumonia*
- *Haemophilus influenza*
- *Moraxella catarrhalis*

If your doctor wants to do a culture, he's trying to identify exactly what bacteria is proliferating to better choose what antibiotic to prescribe.

It may be impossible to determine exactly what combination of bacteria are present, but a culture can be an effective diagnostic tool.

How many times will I have to see my doctor to get my sinusitis cured up?

That's almost impossible to answer. Every case of sinusitis is unique to the individual. Follow your doctor's recommendation and go through the entire course of prescribed treatment, including taking the full course of antibiotics.

How soon will I start to feel better?

In most cases sinusitis begins to resolve in three weeks, but difficult cases can go on for longer. If your symptoms are still present after three months, you have chronic sinusitis, which may mean a long period of trial and error to find the right combination of therapies.

My doctor says I have nasal polyps. How does that affect my sinus problems?

Nasal polyps are simply mucous glands that have become clogged. They are typically about the size of a grape. They are much more common than most people realize, and often burst on their own, with the fluid draining down the throat.

If you've ever had a spontaneous salty taste in the back of your throat, it was probably from a polyp that broke open. Polyps play a role in sinusitis when they block the opening to the sinus and mucus backs up in the chamber.

Under those conditions, bacteria begin to proliferate and lead to an infection. Often polyps will shrink if a course of steroids is used. Occasionally surgical removal is necessary.

How are my allergies connected to my sinusitis?

Allergies cause swelling inside the nasal cavity and can be responsible for blocking the sinuses. If the bacteria in the sinuses then proliferate and an infection develops, then sinusitis is present.

Controlling your allergies may be critical to prevent recurring cases of sinusitis. Often when the two conditions are diagnosed simultaneously your doctor will first work to get the sinusitis in check and then recommend allergy testing and ongoing treatment.

Allergic Rhinitis

What is allergic rhinitis?

Allergic rhinitis and "hay fever" is the same thing. When the affected person breathes in something to which they are sensitive, the body's immune system reacts, causing a series of symptoms including a runny or stuffy nose as well as itching and watering of the eyes.

The sufferer may develop a headache, lose sleep, and have postnasal drip leading to a sore throat. It's also common to temporarily lose the sense of smell.

Common triggers in a bout of allergic rhinitis are pollens, dust mites, mold, fungus spores, and animal dander. It's also possible to be allergic to chemicals and even to perfumes.

These symptoms may occur seasonally, or may only be triggered by accidental exposure. The condition is either treated with a course of desensitizing injections, or with long-term symptom control via prescription or over-the-counter medication.

What causes allergic rhinitis?

When your body is exposed to an allergen, the immune system, for whatever reason, interprets the substance as foreign and a "threat," sending antibodies out to do "war" with the "invader."

The next time you encounter the substance the antibodies essentially recognize it and release histamines to start the fight up again.

In severe cases of allergic rhinitis, the resulting inflammation and irritation leads to other conditions like sinusitis or ear infections. There may even be a link between allergic rhinitis and the development of asthma.

Are there different types of allergic rhinitis?

It's more appropriate to say that there are different "classes" or allergic rhinitis. These designations are based primarily on frequency and severity.

"Intermittent" means the person deals with symptoms on about 4 days a week for less than 4 weeks a year.

"Persistent" indicates 4 or more days for more than 4 weeks, while "mild" indicates symptoms that don't significantly affect sleep patterns or daily activities.

"Moderate to severe" means the symptoms do bother you at home and at work, making normal activities more difficult.

How is allergic rhinitis diagnosed?

Your primary care physician can diagnose allergic rhinitis. Self-diagnosis, however, is quite common and generally safe.

If, however, you are using over-the-counter aids and your symptoms do not improve, or if you begin to experience sinus pain, see your doctor.

Other signs signaling the need for medical intervention include fever, ear pain, a cough that lasts more than 1-2 weeks, and severe itching of the eyes and nose.

What are the treatment options for allergic rhinitis?

Typically whether you see a doctor or treat yourself with over-the-counter products, the mainstays of allergic rhinitis treatment are antihistamines, decongestants, and eye drops.

Note that antihistamines come in "drowsy" and "non-drowsy" variations. Be sure to use the correct one if you don't want to fall asleep at your desk at work!

If OTC remedies don't work, your doctor will be able to prescribe stronger products, including corticosteroid sprays that can provide significant relief of your symptoms.

Be especially careful about OTC nasal decongestants. These products lead to an effect called "rebound" if used for more then 2-3 days. You can become dependent on their decongesting effect.

As soon as the spray wears off, your nose will clog up again, which leads to an even greater use of the product until you literally cannot breathe well without it. The only nasal spray that is safe for use for an extended period of time is plain saline solution.

What are the complications of allergic rhinitis?

The primary complication of allergic rhinitis is the development of sinusitis. Swelling in the nasal passages causes the openings of the sinuses to become blocked. Bacteria proliferate behind the blockage and the area becomes infected.

For someone who has severe allergies, acute and chronic sinusitis is the likely trajectory. Although managing your allergies will help with the sinusitis, once bacterium proliferates, it can be very difficult to effectively eradicate.

Some people with severe allergies also go on to develop asthma, or may be subject to repeated blockages and infections of the Eustachian tubes, which run from the ears to the rear of the throat.

Chronic Sinusitis

How does a deviated septum affect sinusitis?

When the bone and cartilage separating the two sides of the nose is misaligned, you have a "deviated" septum. This condition can itself be responsible for chronic sinusitis, or it can exacerbate sinusitis caused by other problems.

Since most people do have some degree of deviation in the septum, such an irregularity does not always contribute to sinusitis. In chronic cases, however, the state of the septum could be considered.

In severe cases, surgery may be required to straighten the septum. Initially, however, it is recommended that patients try using a nasal strip to open the airway, especially at night.

Nasal strips are adhesive devices that fit across the nose just behind the bulge of the nostrils. They gently widen the nasal vent, that portion of the nose that contracts slightly when we breathe.

Many people with a deviated septum experience the greatest discomfort at night. Sleeping with a nasal strip often relieves this problem in a non-invasive way.

How does asthma affect sinusitis?

In about 30% of cases of acute sinusitis, asthma is also present. The underlying factor in both is constant inflammation, leading to a broader condition of irritation to the mucous membranes in both the nose and lungs referred to as "one airway disease."

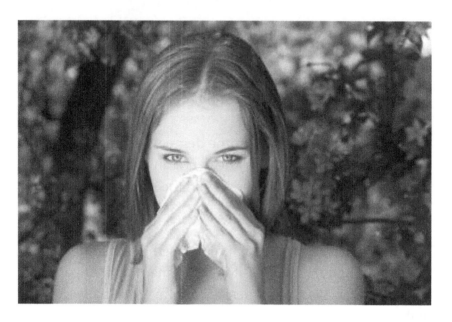

Will allergy shots help to stop my sinus infections?

Allergies can significantly aggravate sinusitis by keep the nasal passages inflamed and clogged, helping to create a breeding ground for bacteria.

Controlling allergies is an important aspect of addressing chronic sinusitis, but the shots are not a quick solution. A series of allergy injections will take 6-24 months to return maximum benefit.

For this reason, long-term allergy treatment should be used in conjunction with other therapies to manage chronic sinusitis. The shots are not a single "solution."

What is the importance of a fungus in sinusitis?

Medical science continues to debate the role of fungus in sinusitis. In a small percentage of cases, fungus is definitely the responsible agent, causing either a "ball" to grow in the sinuses, or contributing to a severe allergic reaction.

In chronic cases of sinusitis, evaluating the potential of a fungal component should be considered as part of a thorough and aggressive evaluation. Surgery is often required in such cases, but the use of antifungal agents and steroids can also be effective.

Will using a vaporizer or humidifier help me?

Humidifiers and vaporizes are very useful especially in the winter when home heating systems drive humidity levels down to 20-30%. The optimum interior humidity for a home is 40-50%.

These units are available in both cold and hot mist varieties. Since it's important not to allow bacteria to grow in the machine itself, the hot mist type that boils the water to create steam is recommended.

Some patients also report gaining additional relief from adding natural decongestants to the water mix like eucalyptus or menthol.

Positioning the vaporizer on your bedside will help to prevent your symptoms from becoming worse overnight.

When should surgery be considered an option?

Surgery should always be considered as the last line treatment for chronic sinusitis. Although this is a challenging condition requiring trial and error therapy, most patients will respond to non-invasive measures to combat their sinusitis.

Estimates vary, but it is believed that in fewer than 10% of cases, sinus surgery is considered a medical necessity. There is always the chance that surgery will not provide the expected relief, which is why all other avenues should be explored first.

What is involved if I do have sinus surgery?

The procedure, called functional endoscopic sinus surgery, requires 2-3 hours and may be performed under either local or general anesthesia.

The operation may involve several types of intervention including realigning a deviated septum, creating openings to enhance drainage, and removing portions of inflamed tissue.

The number of sinuses involved varies by individual. The entire procedure is performed through the nose with the aid of a lighted, magnified endoscope.

Part 5 – Frequently Asked Questions

What is the recovery period following sinus surgery?

In the majority of cases sinus surgery is a day procedure, although some patients may have to stay in the hospital overnight. Most people miss 1-2 weeks of work, with full recovery requiring 6-12 months. During that time, you will be more susceptible to developing sinus infections.

Check-ups will be necessary throughout the recovery to remove any encrusted material to minimize scarring. You will also have to deal with certain prescribed short-term limitations against lifting, blowing your nose, and flying.

After the first week, you will probably be asked to irrigate your nose with saline. There is rarely much if any pain after a nasal procedure, and no external bruising.

Will I still need sinus treatment after surgery?

Sinus surgery is not a guarantee that you will never suffer from sinusitis again. The procedure isn't a cure, only a way to open up your sinuses to facilitate better long-term management of the condition.

It is possible that antibiotics will no longer be required if techniques like nasal irrigation are used with greater effect. Surgery often removes the "hit or miss" element by revealing exactly what's going on in the nasal cavity.

Full access to the area also allows the surgeon to culture portions of the sinus that were previously out of reach for better identification of the bacteria present.

What if the surgery doesn't help at all?

Hard as it may be, it's important to try to be patient after a surgical procedure on the sinuses. A full assessment of the benefits may not be possible for weeks, or even months.

Many factors can contribute to a case of chronic sinusitis, including secondary fungal infections and even autoimmune disease.

Such cases are rare, but in the interest of full disclosure, it's only fair to admit that in some instances, sinus surgery does not make a difference.

Lifestyle and Alternative Treatments

Are there any other non-drug remedies I might try?

Basically, you can try anything that doesn't make your symptoms worse or negatively interact with medications you're taking. Many patients say they derive relief from something as simple as soaking a tissue in eucalyptus oil and breathing in the aroma in concentration throughout the day.

The frequent use of steam from a variety of sources helps hydrate and soothe the sinuses. This can mean frequent hot showers, or steaming under a towel over a bowl of water. For that matter, you can add eucalyptus to the hot water or even apple cider vinegar to heighten the decongesting effect.

Is drinking more water a good idea?

Absolutely. Drinking as much water as possible on a daily basis delivers many positive health effects, not the least of which is thinning of mucus to improve drainage of the sinuses.

Is there any way to completely eliminate sinus infections?

Absolute questions don't beget absolute answers. Particularly in chronic cases of sinusitis, the more you can do to improve your overall health and well-being the greater the chance your future sinus infections will be less frequent and less severe.

Many suffers are satisfied just to reach a point where they do not require as much medication. "Cure" is a more subjective term than you may realize.

Avoiding surgery and having no more than one or two brief flare-ups a year may be as close as some people come to eliminating sinusitis from their lives.

My doctor suggested I start exercising for stress reduction and my sinusitis got worse! Why?

You may actually be suffering from exercise-induced rhinitis or EIR. The most common symptoms are congestion or a runny nose, sneezing, itching/watering eyes/nose, and a postnasal drip.

EIR shows up in both professional and recreational athletes. About 40% of endurance athletes suffer from the condition, which is likely related to breathing in large concentrations of environmental irritants.

The physical exertion places greater oxygen demands on the body. Respiration increases, and with the additional air being taken in along come the irritants.

For the most part the condition is a nuisance, but in people with chronic sinusitis, EIR can make their symptoms worse. You'd do better finding a less strenuous form of exercise until your sinuses improve.

Alternately, you can try using a nasal strip to hold your nasal vent open while you exercise. You may see some football players on TV with these tiny adhesive strips across their noses. This is a simple and effective way to address EIR, and is often the only solution you will require.

Is there really a link between smoking and sinusitis or is my doctor just trying to get me off cigarettes?

While it is certainly possible that your physician would like you to discontinue your use of tobacco products, there is a definite link between cigarette smoking and sinusitis.

When you inhale the smoke from your cigarette, it paralyzes the tiny hairs in your sinus cavities called cilia. They can no longer vibrate to remove mucus and debris.

This allows bacteria to build up in your sinuses so that infection sets in. Once this happens, the ostia or opening to the sinus closes and the area becomes blocked.

Part 5 – Frequently Asked Questions

Afterword

Hopefully you now understand what a marvel of efficiency your sinuses represent when they are open and functioning appropriately, and just how badly everything can fall apart when they're not!

An essential part of the confusion about sinusitis, hay fever, and allergic rhinitis is the indiscrimination with which these terms are mixed and matched.

All represent different points on a spectrum of conditions that can affect how well you are breathing at any given point in time.

Taken singly, each has a unique cause. Typically pollen causes "hay fever" or allergic rhinitis. Bacteria cause sinus infections. Viruses cause colds.

But what happens if you are having your seasonal hay fever, you catch a cold, the combined swelling closes your sinuses, the bacteria build up, and you develop a secondary infection? That's the sinusitis spectrum.

Any of these factors can occur in isolation or all at once, with differing courses of intervention indicated depending on exactly what's going on in your nose, nasal cavity and sinuses.

The challenge is just that – figuring out exactly what's going on. There may be one answer to your problem, or there may be several.

Afterword

A single flare-up of sinusitis may respond quite well to antibiotics, while a chronic case has you playing a game of prescription roulette.

It is imperative that you understand all your options as you grapple with sinusitis in order to make the best treatment decisions. There is, for instance, a common misconception that sinus surgery will "fix" everything.

That is rarely the case. Surgery may improve your condition, but a nasal procedure should not be regarded as a cure and should be a matter of last resort after all other avenues have been explored and exhausted.

Most cases of sinusitis can be resolved or successfully managed, but in a small percentage of cases, the condition is both chronic and stubborn.

Hopefully you will come away from this book with a greater capacity to understand what your doctors are telling you, and to make better choices about your health.

This is the basis of the concept of "informed consent." Never progress with any treatment for any illness until you fully understand what is being recommended and all associated ramifications.

Keep asking questions, and don't stop until you get all the answers you need!

Especially with the potential for a chronic condition that may be a part of your life for several years, your goal is to

Afterword

be a participant in your own health care, not a patient who simply does as they are told.

After all, you have to live with your sinusitis – and with the consequences of any "cure" you try.

Afterword

Relevant Websites

American Academy of Allergy Asthma & Immunology
www.aaaai.org/conditions-and-
treatments/allergies/sinusitis.aspx

University of Maryland Medical Center
www.umm.edu/health/medical/reports/articles/sinusitis

Centers for Disease Control and Prevention
www.cdc.gov/getsmart/antibiotic-use/uri/sinus-
infection.html

Harvard Health Publications
www.health.harvard.edu/books/Healing_Your_Sinuses

The John Hopkins Sinus Center
www.hopkinsmedicine.org/sinus/sinus_conditions/rhinosi
nusitis.html

Healthy Children
www.healthychildren.org/English/health-
issues/conditions/ear-nose-throat/pages/The-Difference-
Between-Sinusitis-and-a-Cold.aspx

The Mayo Clinic
http://www.mayoclinic.com/health/chronic-
sinusitis/DS00232

Relevant Websites

Glossary

A

acute sinusitis - In cases of acute sinusitis, symptoms last more than a few weeks, but less than three months.

allergic rhinitis - A series of nasal symptoms generated by a reaction to an allergen. The response typically includes congestion / runny nose, headache, sneezing, and watering / itching eyes. Also called "hay fever."

allergy - An adverse physical reaction to given environmental irritants, which may include pollens, fungus, foods, or microorganisms. The immune system responds with a series of measures intended to drive off the "invader," which may include sneezing, nasal congestion, and itching. An allergic reaction is often a precursor to an attack of sinusitis.

amoxicillin - An antibiotic that is a variant of penicillin and is the most frequently prescribed medication for sinus infections.

antibody - Molecules used by the immune system in an attempt to combat "invading" substances like allergens, bacteria, or viruses.

B

bromelain - A natural compound found in pineapples that reputedly reduces the symptoms of sinusitis.

C

cephalosporin - A class of antibiotics used in treatment of sinusitis as an alternative to the penicillins.

chronic sinusitis - A case of sinusitis with a duration of more than three months. The most difficult type of sinusitis to treat.

cilia - Tiny hairs present in the lining of the sinuses that normally vibrate for the purpose of removing mucus and expelling any debris present.

concha bullosa - A term describing the enlargement of the middle turbinate that may lead to an obstruction of the sinuses.

cogeners - By-products of the fermentation process found in alcoholic beverages that may trigger sinusitis symptoms in some people.

CT scan - The accepted acronym for computed tomography, a form of x-ray that generates a series of cross sections of a body structure to generate a three-dimensional image. Considered to be the best method for diagnosing nasal abnormalities in cases of sinusitis.

D

deviated septum - A misalignment of the nasal septum separating the nostrils. May be responsible for blocking

---

breathing and causing the congestion present in chronic sinusitis.

E

endoscope - A high-resolution telescope thin enough to be inserted in the nose for diagnostic and surgical purposes.

ENT doctor - The acronym for "ear, nose, and throat." Doctors that specialize in ailments in these areas are properly called otolaryngologists.

ethmoid sinuses - The pair of multi-chambered sinuses located between the eyes.

Eustachian tubes - The tube leading from the ears to the back of the throat, which serves to equalize pressure in the ears.

F

FESS - Nasal surgery using an endoscope in the nostrils to allow for visualization of the nasal cavity and sinuses.

frontal sinus drillout - A surgical procedure for the removal of the floor of the frontal sinus to improve mucus drainage.

frontal sinuses - The sinuses located in the forehead.

fungal ball sinusitis - A form of sinusitis caused by the proliferation of fungus in the sinus cavity that grows into a mass shaped like a ball. Typically occurs in the maxillary sinuses.

G

guaifenesin - The active ingredient found in medications that serve to thin mucus secretions.

I

invasive fungal sinusitis - An extremely rare form of sinusitis caused by fungus that invades the wall of the sinuses reaching the bone and blood vessels and potentially spreading to the brain. Often occurs in people with severely impaired immune systems.

L

lamina papyracea - The paper thin segment of bone separating the eye socket from the ethmoid sinus.

M

macrolide - The class of antibiotic typically prescribed to patients that exhibit an allergic reaction to penicillin.

magnetic resonance imaging (MRI) - A radiological technique most appropriate for visualizing soft tissues in the body. Ineffective for imaging the sinuses.

maxillary sinuses - The sinuses found in the cheekbones that extend from just under the eyes to the region above the upper teeth.

migraine - Recurrent, severe headaches that can be mistaken for sinus pain but that constitute a completely different condition.

mucociliary clearance - The process by which the cilia in the sinuses sweep mucus and debris from the cavity during normal daily drainage.

mucous membrane - Sheets of tissue that line the nose and sinuses (among other structures in the body). The glands in the tissue secrete mucus.

mucus - This substance, excreted by the mucous membranes in the nose and sinuses, moisturizes the structures and serves to trap foreign particles and debris.

N

nasal cycle - Every six hours, breathing switches sides on the nose so that each is alternately dominant. A normal occurrence often mistaken as a sinusitis symptom.

nasal lavage - A term for rinsing or irrigating the nasal cavity.

nasal septum - The partition of bone and cartilage that separates the two sides of the nose. Roughly three inches in length.

nasal steroids - Anti-inflammatory drugs used for the purpose of reducing swelling in the nasal cavity and sinuses. Available in spray and pill form.

nasal tape - An adhesive strip sold over-the-counter for the purpose of temporarily widening the nasal valve to improve breathing.

nasal valve - The middle third of the nose just above the bulge of the nostrils that moves slightly as we inhale and exhale.

neti pot - A small cup with a handle and spout used for effective nasal irrigation.

neuralgia - Nerve pain that affects the face and may be mistaken for a case of sinusitis.

neuritis - A condition involving inflammation of nerve endings. When neuritis occurs in the face, it can be mistaken for sinusitis

O

ostiomeatal complex (OMC) - Narrow channels that serve as a point of drainage for the ethmoid, maxillary, and frontal sinuses. Obstruction of this area is a common cause of sinusitis.
otolaryngologist - A doctor commonly referred to as an ENT that specializes in diseases of the ears, nose, and throat.

P

pansinusitis - A case of sinusitis involving infections of all four pairs of sinuses.

phlegm - An alternate term for a collection of mucus in the back of the throat. Typical in a case of sinusitis, especially in the morning.

polyp - Growths in the sinuses that are roughly the size of a grape. Often present in patients with chronic inflammation. May obstruct the nasal passages causing sinusitis and impairing breathing.

pseudoephedrine - The active ingredient found in oral decongestants.

pus - Yellow or green liquid present in infections that often drains into the sinuses and down the throat. Contains the mass of white blood cells dispensed by the immune system for the purpose of fighting infection.

Q

quinolones - The most powerful class of antibiotics typically used for the most difficult and persistent sinus infections.

R

rebound - A negative consequence of over-using nasal sprays signaling dependence on the medication. When a dose is not administered, the symptoms of congestion return instantly and with greater severity.

revision surgery - Any surgery performed as a follow-up or corrective measure subsequent to an initial surgery.

rhinitis - A term describing inflammation of the mucous membranes of the nose and sinsuses.

sinusitis - A condition characterized by inflammation of the sinuses.

sphenoid sinuses - The sinuses located behind the nose.

T

triad asthma - A type of asthma present in some cases of chronic sinusitis marked by asthma, the presence of nasal polyps, and an allergic reaction to aspirin. Also called Samter's triad or aspirin-induced asthma.

turbinates - Bones inside the nose that are scroll-shaped and covered by mucous membranes. They serve to condition and moisten air before it reaches the lungs.

V

vacuum sinusitis - A type of sinusitis in which the lining of a blocked sinus absorbs oxygen. This causes a painful vacuum (negative pressure) to form in the sinus.

Index

abscesses, 46, 85

acetaminophen, 61

Allergic fungal sinusitis, 52

allergic reaction, 49, 67, 97

allergic rhinitis, 2, 15, 16, 38, 47, 50, 91, 92, 93, 94, 105

allergies, 13

amoxicillin, 42, 63, 65, 66, 85, 86

animal dander, 15, 91

antihistamines, 58, 60, 87, 93

aspirin, 40, 49, 61

asthma, 49, 95

augmentin, 42, 63

autoimmune disorder, 47

azelastine, 61

Azelastine, 61

azithromycin, 42, 64, 66, 86

bacteria, 14, 22, 24, 25, 26

Bacteroides, 65

bad breath, 30, 32, *See* halitosis

blood, 19, 25

blood vessels, 53

Broad spectrum antibiotics, 67

bromphenirmaine, 60

bruising, 63, 70, 99

carbon dioxide, 16

carotid artery, 22

carpeting, 15

cartilage, 17, 95

cataracts, 63

cefdinir, 42, 64, 66, 86

cefixime, 66

cefpodoxime, 42, 64, 66, 86

cefuroxime, 66

cephalexin, 66

cephalosporins, 65, 66

cetirizine, 60

chlorpheniramine, 60

cilia, 22, 24

ciprofloxacin, 67

clarithromycin, 42, 64, 66, 86

clavulanate, 42, 63, 85

clemastine, 60

common cold, 13, 14

congestion, 20, 28, 29, 32, 37, 43, 45, 49, 50, 51, 71, 76, 77, 78, 102

Corticosteroid sprays, 61

cough, 30, 58, 59, 84, 93

-cough medicine, 58

cranial cavity, 23

culture, 38, 39, 65, 88, 99

decongestant, 34, 35, 42, 43, 59, 86

Index

Index

Lightning Source UK Ltd.
Milton Keynes UK
UKOW06f2323130416

272213UK00018B/330/P